MOTHER NATURE IS TRYING TO KILL ME!

DEADLY DISEASES

BY JANEY LEVY

Gareth Stevens
PUBLISHING

Please visit our website, www.garethstevens.com. For a free color catalog of all our high-quality books, call toll free 1-800-542-2595 or fax 1-877-542-2596.

Library of Congress Cataloging-in-Publication Data

Names: Levy, Janey, author.
Title: Deadly diseases / Janey Levy.
Description: New York : Gareth Stevens Publishing, [2020] | Series: Mother nature is trying to kill me! | Includes index.
Identifiers: LCCN 2018044074| ISBN 9781538239629 (paperback) | ISBN 9781538239643 (library bound) | ISBN 9781538239636 (6 pack)
Subjects: LCSH: Communicable diseases–Juvenile literature. | Epidemics–Juvenile literature.
Classification: LCC RA643 .L48 2020 | DDC 616.9–dc23
LC record available at https://lccn.loc.gov/2018044074

First Edition

Published in 2020 by
Gareth Stevens Publishing
111 East 14th Street, Suite 349
New York, NY 10003

Copyright © 2020 Gareth Stevens Publishing

Designer: Sarah Liddell
Editor: Monika Davies

Photo credits: Cover, p. 1 Sebastian Kaulitzki/Shutterstock.com; background used throughout Jezper/Shutterstock.com; p. 4 krumanop/Shutterstock.com; p. 5 yochika photographer/Shutterstock.com; p. 7 (main) Chaikom/Shutterstock.com; p. 7 (inset) Festa/Shutterstock.com; p. 9 (main) Tacio Philip Sansonovski/Shutterstock.com; p. 9 (inset), 11 (inset) Kateryna Kon/Shutterstock.com; p. 11 (main) JEKESAI NJIKIZANA/AFP/Getty Images; p. 13 Thierry Falise/Contributor/LightRocket/Getty Images; p. 15 Boston Globe/Contributor/Boston Globe/Getty Images; p. 17 (main) Suwannee Ngoenklan/Shutterstock.com; p. 17 (inset) Ezume Images/Shutterstock.com; p. 19 (main) FAYEZ NURELDINE/Staff/AFP/Getty Images; p. 19 (inset) Nixx Photography/Shutterstock.com; p. 20 TinnaPong/Shutterstock.com; p. 21 Christoph Burgstedt/Shutterstock.com.

All rights reserved. No part of this book may be reproduced in any form without permission in writing from the publisher, except by a reviewer.

Printed in the United States of America

CPSIA compliance information: Batch #CS19GS: For further information contact Gareth Stevens, New York, New York at 1-800-542-2595.

CONTENTS

Death-Dealing Diseases 4
Evil Ebola 6
Dangerous Dengue 8
Killer Cholera 10
Menacing Malaria 12
Nasty Necrotizing Fasciitis 14
Murderous Meningitis 16
Monstrous MERS 18
Fighting Back 20
Glossary 22
For More Information 23
Index 24

Words in the glossary appear in **bold** type
the first time they are used in the text.

DEATH-DEALING DISEASES

Disease, or illness, is something everyone deals with. You likely get a cold at least once a year. Most of the time, the diseases we get are nothing dangerous. They're bothersome, but nothing worse. But some diseases are deadly!

Some of the world's deadliest diseases kill in especially horrible ways. This can cause much suffering for **victims**. These diseases can kill quickly—sometimes in just a few hours! Some of these diseases have existed for centuries, while others have only recently appeared.

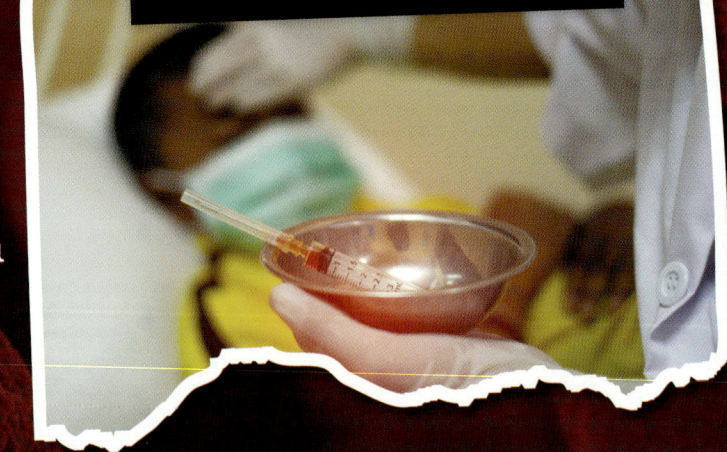

DEADLY DISEASES CAN BE HIGHLY CONTAGIOUS, WHICH MEANS THEY'RE PASSED EASILY FROM PERSON TO PERSON.

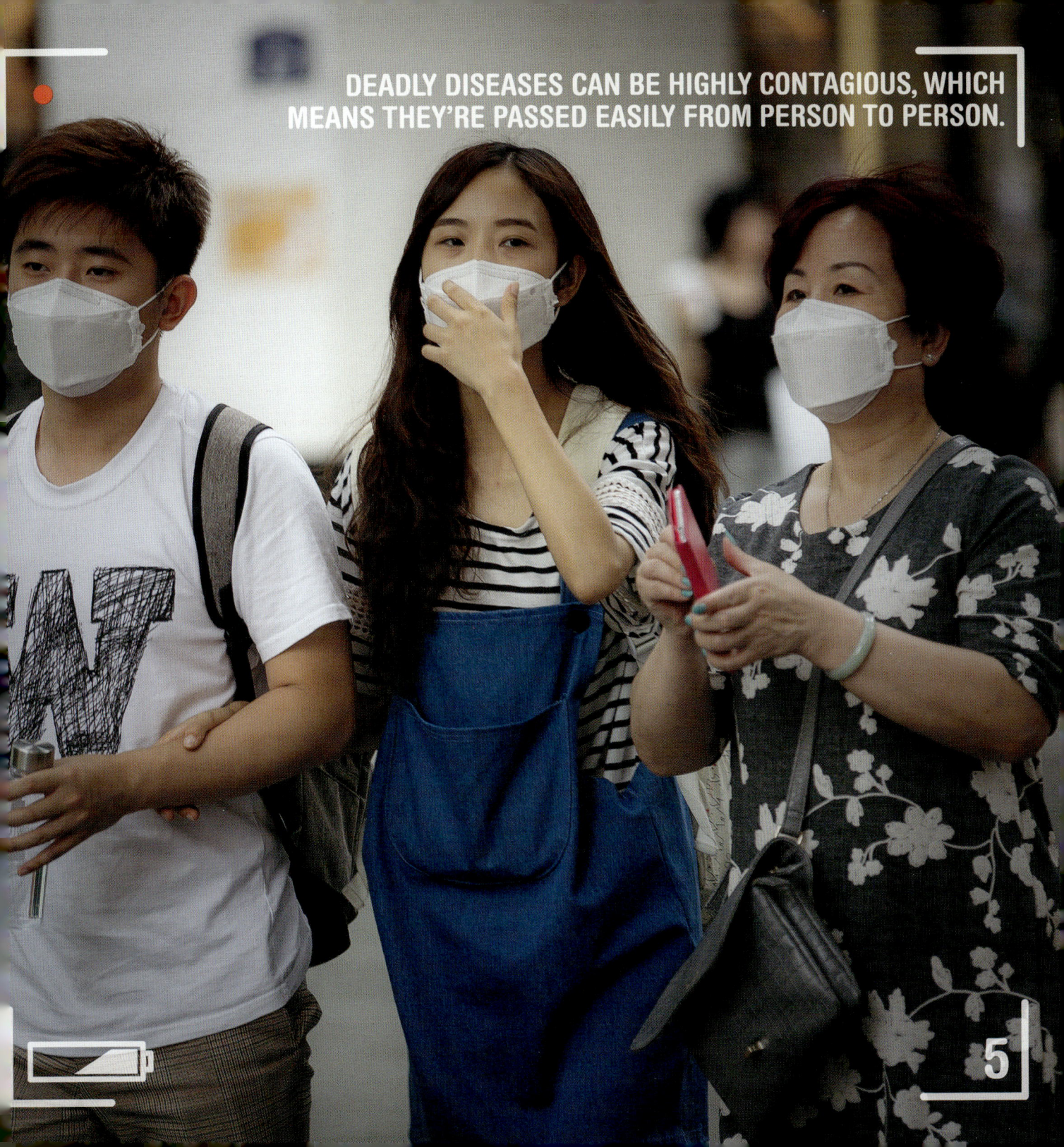

5

EVIL EBOLA

Ebola was named after Africa's Ebola River, where it was first discovered in 1976. It's one of the scariest and deadliest diseases in the world.

If you get Ebola, it first feels like you might have the flu. You feel tired, and your **muscles,** head, and throat hurt. You start to develop a fever and may begin throwing up. Then, it gets much worse. You begin bleeding, often from your eyes or mouth, as well as inside your body. Death usually comes quickly after that.

THE FORCE OF NATURE

ON AVERAGE, EBOLA KILLS ABOUT HALF OF THE PEOPLE WHO ARE INFECTED. AT ITS WORST, IT CAN KILL UP TO 90 PERCENT OF THE PEOPLE INFECTED!

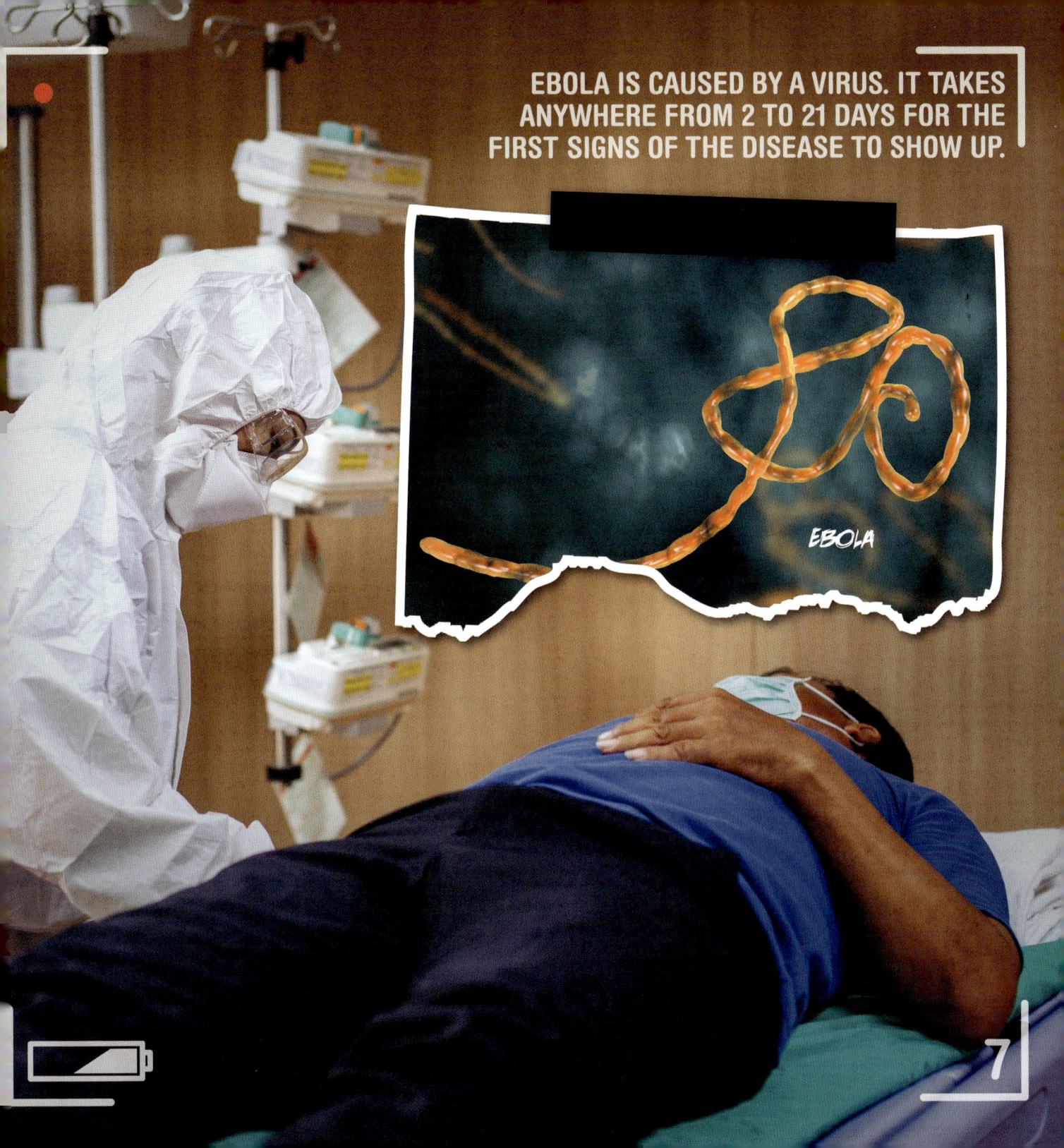

EBOLA IS CAUSED BY A VIRUS. IT TAKES ANYWHERE FROM 2 TO 21 DAYS FOR THE FIRST SIGNS OF THE DISEASE TO SHOW UP.

EBOLA

Dangerous Dengue

Dengue is a disease caused by a virus you get from a **mosquito** bite. Most of the time, people with dengue have a harmless, flu-like sickness. But, on rare occasions, dengue can turn deadly.

The flu-like dengue may become a hemorrhagic, or bleeding, disease. You might feel very tired and have trouble breathing. Blood may come out of your nose or mouth, and you might begin throwing up blood. As with Ebola, it's a terrible way to die.

The Force of Nature

The hemorrhagic form of dengue can kill within hours. If untreated, up to 20 percent of people with the disease die.

THE DENGUE VIRUS HAS ONLY BEEN FOUND IN CERTAIN AREAS OF THE WORLD, INCLUDING PARTS OF SOUTHEAST ASIA, AUSTRALIA, AND AFRICA.

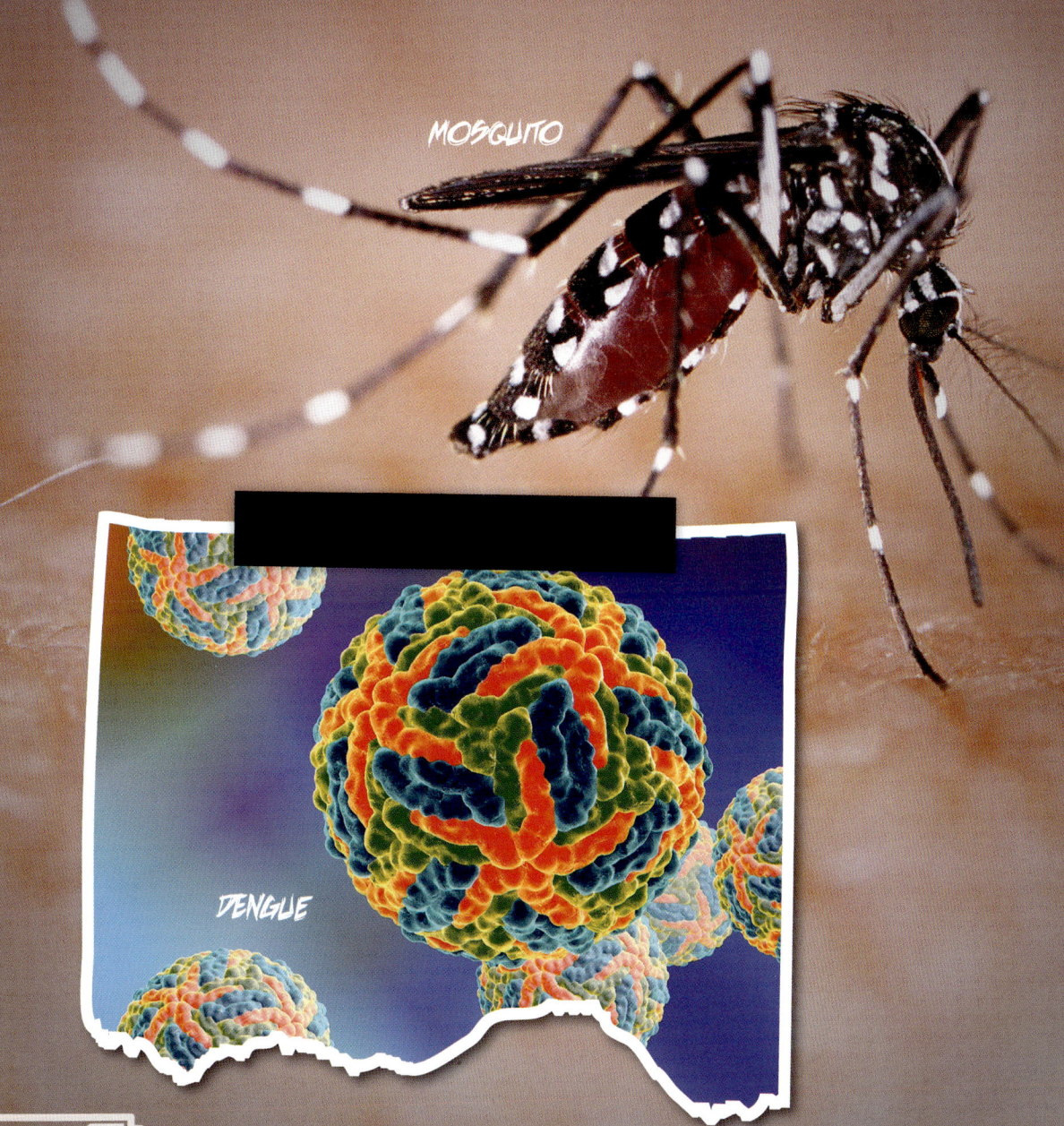

MOSQUITO

DENGUE

KILLER CHOLERA

Cholera is caused by a **bacterium**. If you're very lucky, you might have no **symptoms** when you have cholera. If you're partially lucky, you may only have mild diarrhea, or very soft or runny solid waste. However, in severe cases, the disease can take your life.

Cholera causes **extreme**, watery diarrhea. It makes you throw up. Your body loses so much water that you become very **dehydrated**, as if you were lost in the desert without water. This can lead to death.

> **THE FORCE OF NATURE**
>
> IN 2016, THERE WERE OVER 132,000 CASES OF CHOLERA AROUND THE WORLD. MORE THAN 2,400 PEOPLE DIED FROM THE DISEASE.

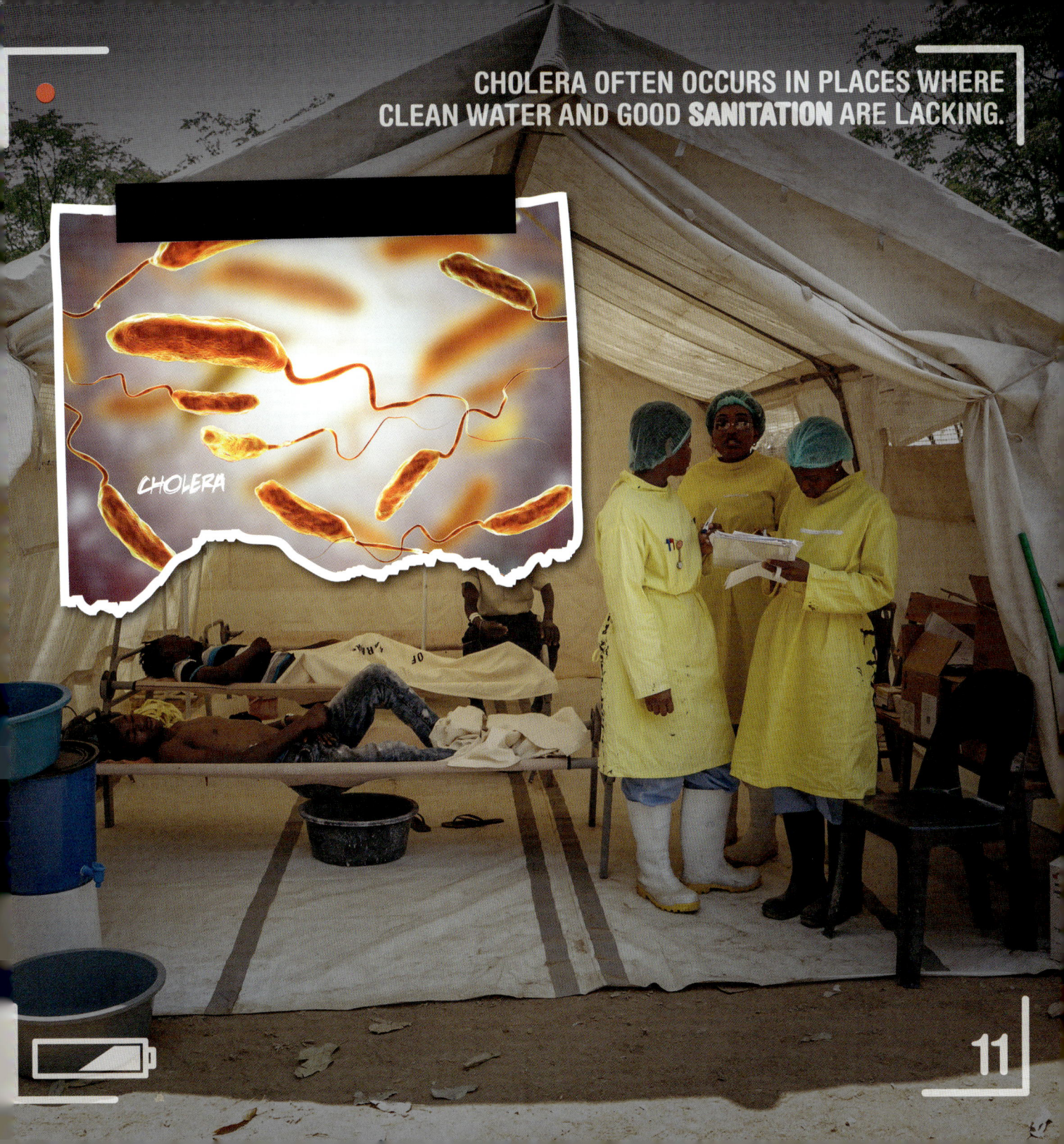

CHOLERA OFTEN OCCURS IN PLACES WHERE CLEAN WATER AND GOOD **SANITATION** ARE LACKING.

CHOLERA

MENACING MALARIA

Malaria is caused by a parasite, which is passed to humans through the bite of an infected mosquito. A parasite is a living thing that lives in, on, or with another living thing and often harms it.

If you get malaria, you'll usually have a high fever and sweat a lot. At the same time, you might shiver and feel chilly. When malaria gets really bad, your brain may start to swell. **Organs** inside your body may begin to fail. These effects can cause death.

THE FORCE OF NATURE

MALARIA IS THE CAUSE OF DEATH FOR OVER 400,000 PEOPLE EACH YEAR. BABIES AND YOUNG CHILDREN ARE OFTEN THE MOST LIKELY TO GET BAD CASES OF MALARIA.

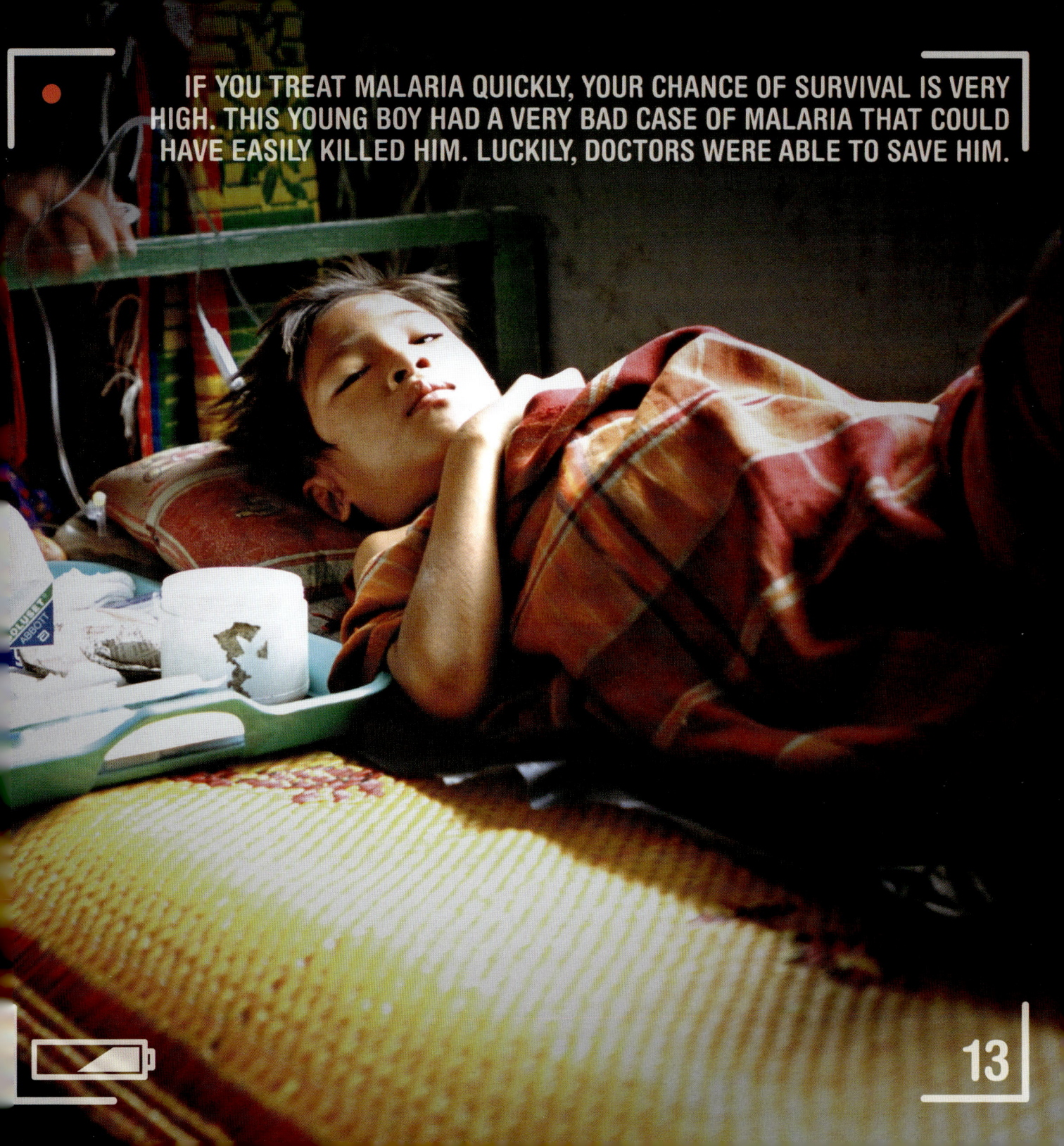

IF YOU TREAT MALARIA QUICKLY, YOUR CHANCE OF SURVIVAL IS VERY HIGH. THIS YOUNG BOY HAD A VERY BAD CASE OF MALARIA THAT COULD HAVE EASILY KILLED HIM. LUCKILY, DOCTORS WERE ABLE TO SAVE HIM.

NASTY NECROTIZING FASCIITIS

Necrotizing fasciitis is better known by a more popular name: flesh-eating bacteria. Flesh-eating bacteria sounds scary—and it is!

Several types of bacteria cause this disease. The bacteria enter your body through a break in the skin, such as a cut. Then, the bacteria quickly go to work. They destroy the matter that surrounds muscles and other body parts under the skin. It's hard to stop these bacteria, and doctors often must cut off sufferers' arms or legs. Even then, people often die.

THE FORCE OF NATURE

WHILE THE CHANCES OF GETTING FLESH-EATING BACTERIA IS VERY LOW, AROUND 700 TO 1,200 PEOPLE IN THE UNITED STATES ARE INFECTED EACH YEAR. AROUND ONE IN FOUR PEOPLE INFECTED DIE.

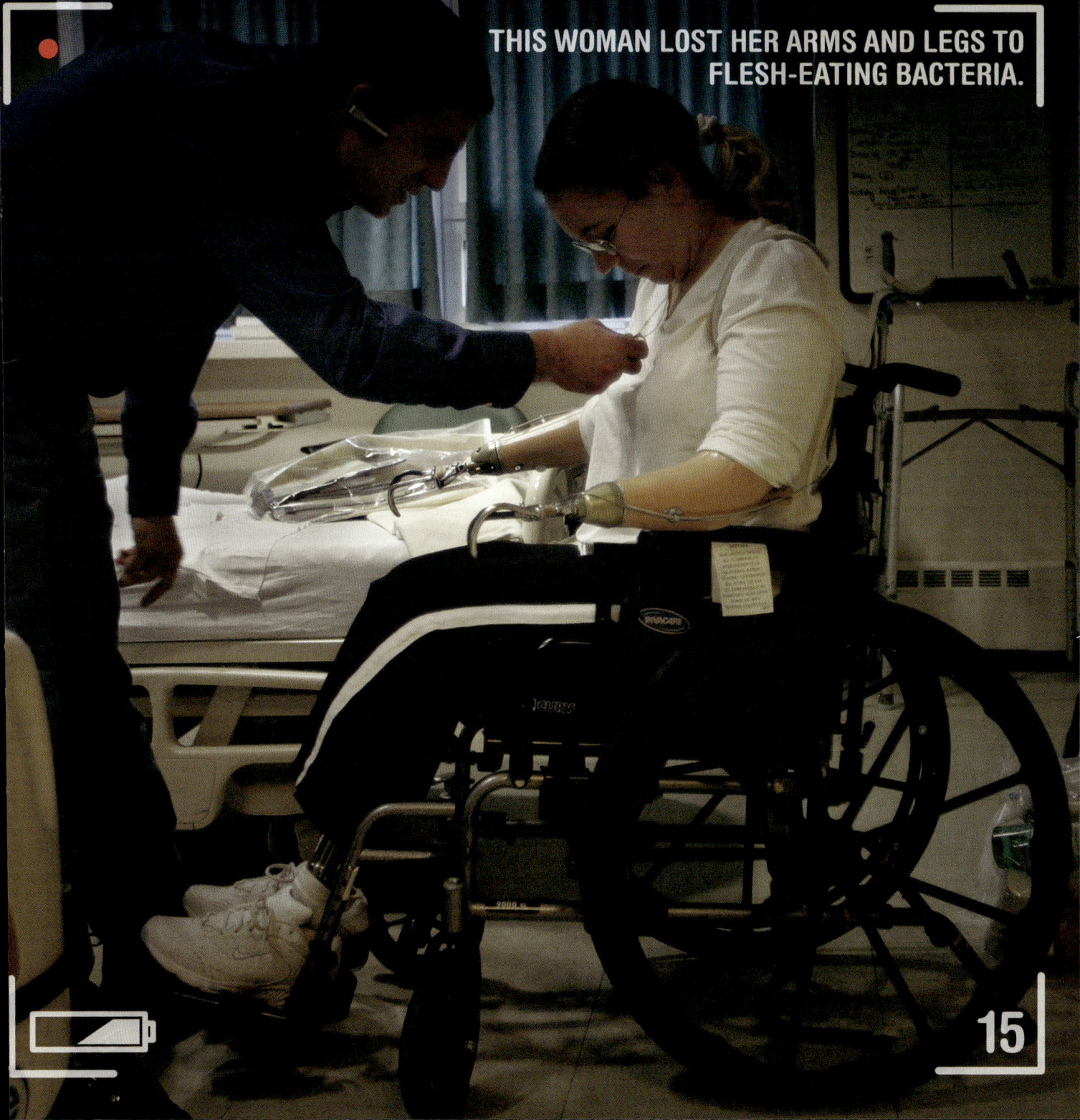

THIS WOMAN LOST HER ARMS AND LEGS TO FLESH-EATING BACTERIA.

15

MURDEROUS MENINGITIS

Meningitis is a swelling of the meninges, or coverings, around your brain and spinal cord. Anything that acts on your brain must be terrifying!

Meningitis is often caused by bacteria or a virus. Symptoms include a sudden high fever, stiff neck, and very bad head pain. You may throw up and become sleepy. Thinking and walking could become difficult. You might get blood poisoning and wind up having your arms or legs cut off. You may also suffer lasting brain harm—or end up dead.

THE FORCE OF NATURE

THE BACTERIA THAT CAUSES BACTERIAL MENINGITIS CAN PASS FROM PERSON TO PERSON. FOR EXAMPLE, THE DISEASE CAN SPREAD WHEN AN INFECTED PERSON COUGHS AND ANOTHER BREATHES IN THAT AIR.

WHILE MENINGITIS IS A DEADLY DISEASE, MANY YOUNG PEOPLE ARE **IMMUNE** TO THE DISEASE BECAUSE THEY'VE RECEIVED THE MENINGOCOCCAL VACCINE. VACCINES ARE SHOTS THAT KEEP A PERSON FROM GETTING CERTAIN DISEASES, SUCH AS MENINGITIS.

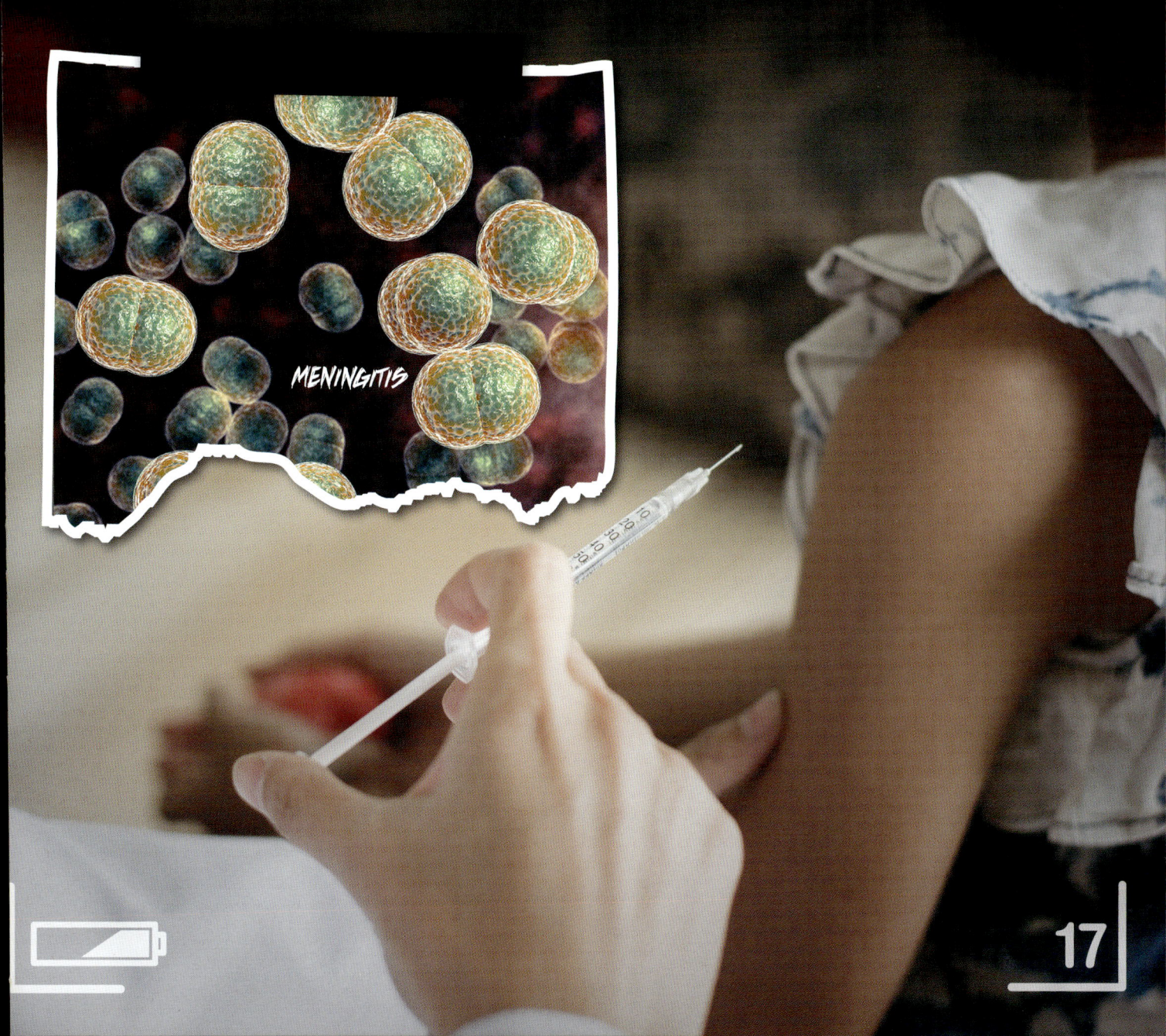

MENINGITIS

MONSTROUS MERS

"MERS" stands for Middle East **Respiratory** Syndrome. This disease harms the respiratory system, or the group of organs that helps you breathe.

MERS is caused by the same kind of virus that causes colds. If you get the MERS virus, you might have symptoms that seem very similar to having a cold. However, your symptoms can become much worse. You may have a fever and cough, as well as have trouble breathing. You might throw up and have diarrhea. Many people have died from MERS.

THE FORCE OF NATURE

THE MERS VIRUS FIRST APPEARED IN SAUDI ARABIA IN 2012. THE DISEASE THEN SPREAD TO OTHER COUNTRIES. AROUND 30 PERCENT OF PEOPLE WITH MERS DIE.

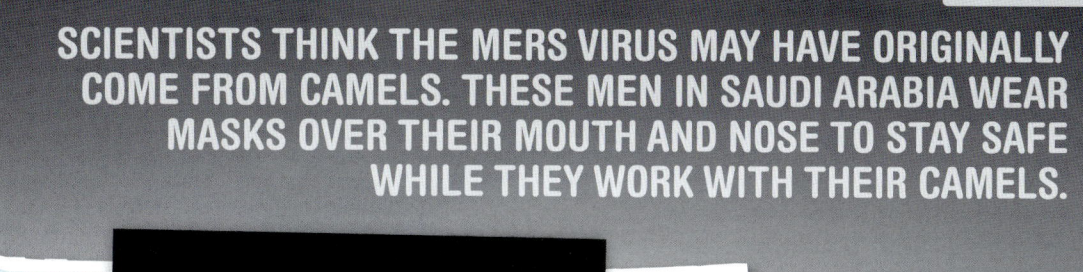

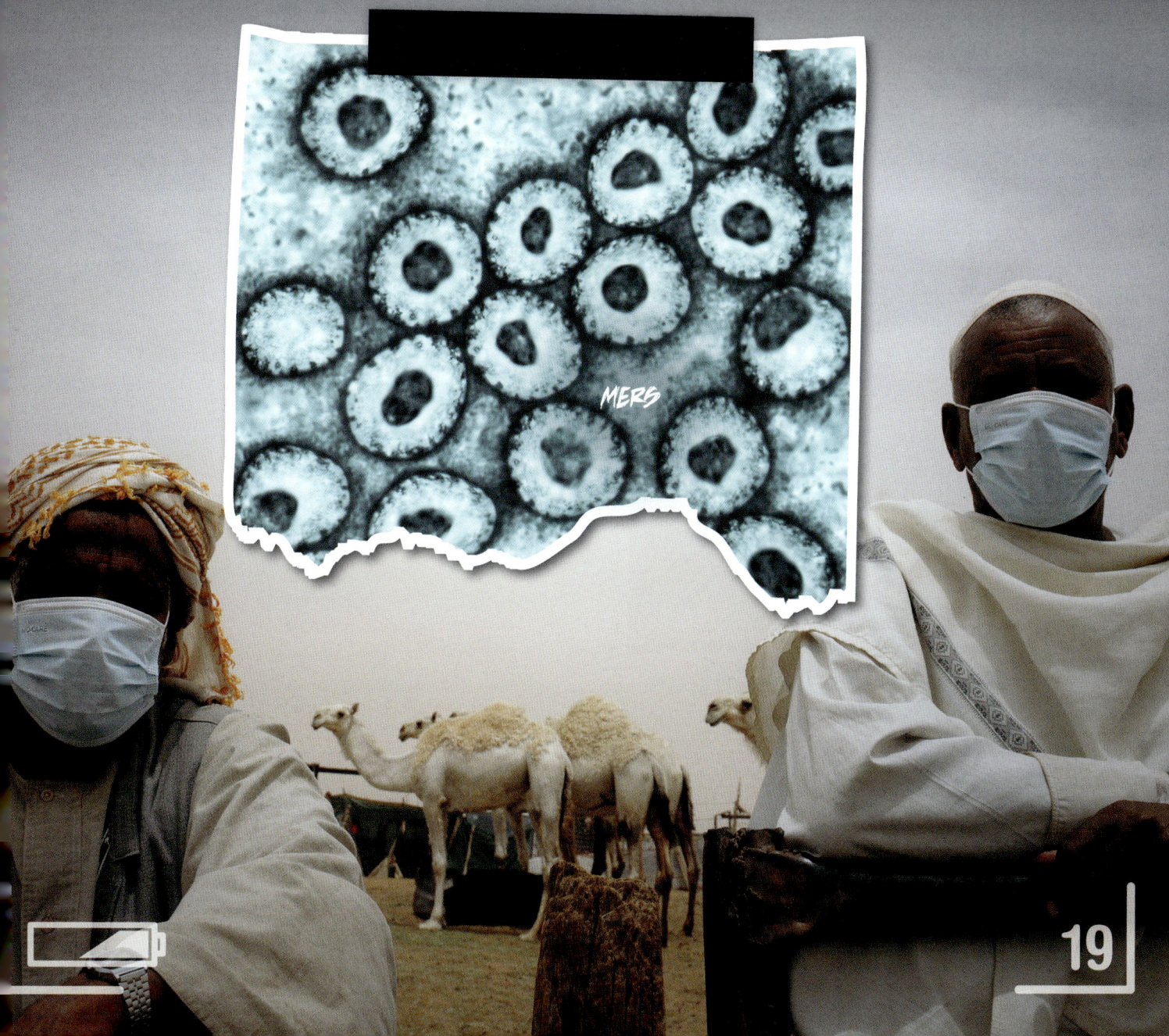

SCIENTISTS THINK THE MERS VIRUS MAY HAVE ORIGINALLY COME FROM CAMELS. THESE MEN IN SAUDI ARABIA WEAR MASKS OVER THEIR MOUTH AND NOSE TO STAY SAFE WHILE THEY WORK WITH THEIR CAMELS.

MERS

FIGHTING BACK

In a world filled with horrible diseases, what keeps us safe? Scientists are always looking for new ways to treat deadly diseases. They've found ways to treat some diseases, including malaria and cholera.

However, the best methods to stay healthy are sometimes up to you. Use bug spray to prevent mosquito bites. Wash your hands often. If you have symptoms of a deadly disease, go see your doctor immediately for treatment. You can fight back!

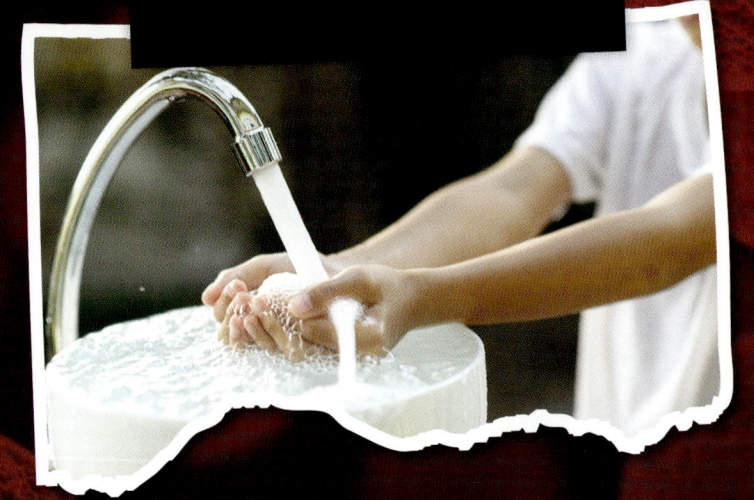

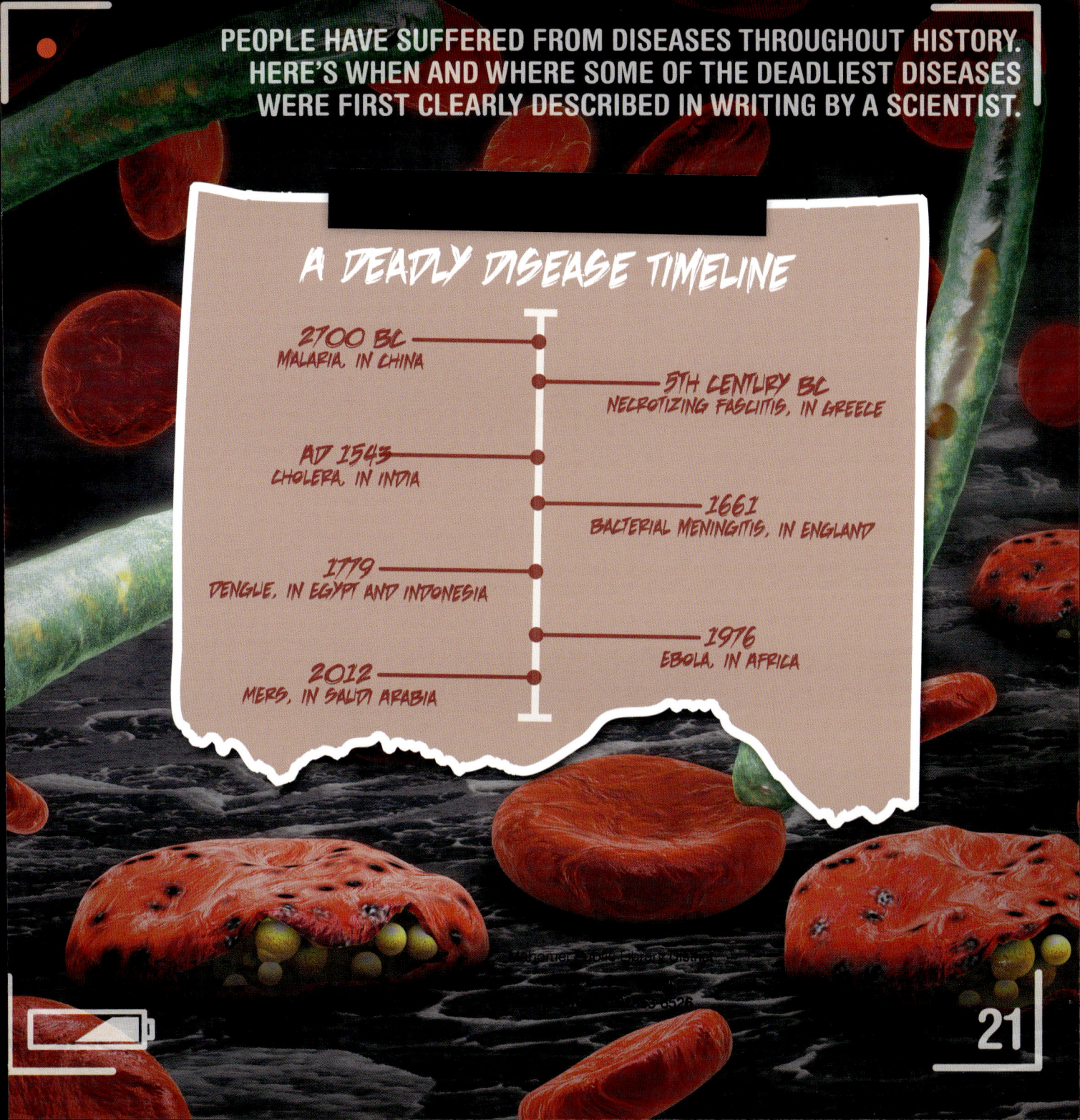

PEOPLE HAVE SUFFERED FROM DISEASES THROUGHOUT HISTORY. HERE'S WHEN AND WHERE SOME OF THE DEADLIEST DISEASES WERE FIRST CLEARLY DESCRIBED IN WRITING BY A SCIENTIST.

A DEADLY DISEASE TIMELINE

- **2700 BC** — Malaria, in China
- **5th century BC** — Necrotizing Fasciitis, in Greece
- **AD 1543** — Cholera, in India
- **1661** — Bacterial Meningitis, in England
- **1779** — Dengue, in Egypt and Indonesia
- **1976** — Ebola, in Africa
- **2012** — MERS, in Saudi Arabia

GLOSSARY

bacterium: a tiny creature that can only be seen with a microscope. The plural is bacteria.

dehydrated: when too much water is lost

extreme: great or severe

immune: not able to get a certain disease

mosquito: a small fly that feeds on the blood of some animals and can spread illness

muscle: one of the parts of the body that allow movement

organ: a part inside an animal's body

respiratory: having to do with the body's organs used to breathe

sanitation: having to do with actions taken for health and cleanliness

symptom: a change or sign that shows someone is sick or unwell

victim: a person who has been hurt

FOR MORE INFORMATION

BOOKS

Arnold, Nick. *Horrible Science: Deadly Diseases*. London, England: Scholastic, 2014.

Ford, Jeanne Marie. *Malaria: How a Parasite Changed History*. North Mankato, MN: Capstone Press, 2019.

Squire, Ann O. *Ebola*. New York, NY: Children's Press, 2016.

WEBSITES

BAM! Body and Mind
www.cdc.gov/bam/diseases/index.html
Become a "disease detective" and go hunting through the CDC's database to learn more about a variety of common diseases.

Ebola
kidshealth.org/en/kids/ebola.html
Learn what exactly Ebola is, how people get the disease, where it came from, and more!

Pandemic Flu . . . What to Do, What to Do!
kids.niehs.nih.gov/topics/healthy-living/pandemic-flu/index.htm
Discover what a pandemic flu is, and learn how to stay healthy and be prepared!

Publisher's note to educators and parents: Our editors have carefully reviewed these websites to ensure that they are suitable for students. Many websites change frequently, however, and we cannot guarantee that a site's future contents will continue to meet our high standards of quality and educational value. Be advised that students should be closely supervised whenever they access the internet.

INDEX

Africa 6, 9, 21
bacteria 10, 14, 16
bleeding 6, 8
brain 12, 16
breathing trouble 8, 18
camels 19
cholera 10, 11, 20, 21
dehydration 10
dengue 8, 9, 21
diarrhea 10, 18
Ebola 6, 7, 8, 21
fever 6, 12, 16, 18
flesh-eating bacteria 14, 15
flu 6, 8
malaria 12, 13, 20, 21

meningitis 16, 17, 21
MERS 18, 19, 21
mosquitos 8, 9, 12, 20
necrotizing fasciitis 14, 21
organ failure 12
parasites 12
respiratory system 18
sanitation 11
Saudi Arabia 18, 19, 21
throwing up 6, 8, 10, 16, 18
tiredness 6, 8, 16
United States 14
vaccines 17
virus 7, 8, 9, 16, 18